# OPTIMIZE YOUR HEALTH WITH ANIMAL-BASED FOOD

# 101 RECIPES

## BY

# DAPHNE E HOWARD

# TABLE OF CONTENT

# INTRODUCTION

In recent years, the conversation surrounding nutrition has become increasingly complex, with various dietary philosophies and trends emerging. Amidst this plethora of information, one approach that has stood the test of time and garnered considerable attention is the consumption of animal-based foods for optimal health and well-being.

The notion of optimizing health through animal-based foods harks back to ancestral diets, where our predecessors relied on a diverse array of animal products for sustenance and vitality. From nutrient-dense meats and fish to nourishing dairy products and eggs, these foods provided essential nutrients crucial for growth, development, and overall vitality.

In this modern age, where dietary choices abound, the significance of animal-based foods remains undeniable. They serve as rich sources of high-quality protein, essential amino acids, vitamins, and minerals vital for supporting various bodily functions, including muscle growth, immune function, and cognitive health. Moreover, animal-based foods offer a unique combination of nutrients that are often more bioavailable and readily absorbed by the body compared to plant-based alternatives. This bioavailability ensures that our bodies can efficiently utilize the nutrients present in these foods, maximizing their health-promoting benefits.

However, the consumption of animal-based foods is not without controversy, as ethical, environmental, and health concerns have fueled debates surrounding their place in a balanced diet. While these concerns warrant consideration and discussion, it's essential to recognize that responsibly sourced animal products can be part of a sustainable and healthful dietary pattern.

In this series, we will delve into the myriad benefits of incorporating animal-based foods into your diet while addressing common misconceptions and concerns. From exploring the nutritional profile of different animal products to discussing practical tips for sourcing high-quality options, we aim to empower you to make informed dietary choices that support your health and well-being.
Ultimately, whether you choose to embrace a predominantly animal-based diet or incorporate these foods alongside plant-based options, the key lies in prioritizing nutrient-density, quality, and balance. By understanding the role of animal-based foods in

optimizing health and making conscious choices that align with your individual needs and values, you can embark on a journey toward vitality and wellness that is both satisfying and sustainable.

# CHAPTER 1
# ANIMAL-BASED NUTRITION

Consuming foods that are derived from animal sources in order to fulfill the nutritional requirements of the body is what is meant by the term "animal-based nutrition." Meat, poultry, fish, eggs, dairy products, and other products derived from animals are included in this category of nutritious foods. Protein, vitamins (especially B12), minerals (like iron and calcium), and healthy fats (like omega-3 fatty acids) are some of the essential nutrients that can be obtained from animal-based nutrition. It is an essential component in the maintenance of a wide range of bodily functions, including the development and repair of muscles, the regulation of hormones, the functioning of the immune system, and overall health. Consuming an excessive amount of foods derived from animals, on the other hand, has been linked to a number of health problems, including cardiovascular diseases, obesity, and certain types of cancer. For this reason, it is absolutely necessary to always consume a well-balanced diet that consists of both plant-based and animal-based foods in order to guarantee the best possible nutrition and health. These essential macronutrients include protein and fats, as well as essential micronutrients such as vitamins (especially B12), minerals (such as iron and calcium), and essential fatty acids (such as omega-3s). Animal-based nutrition is a source of these essential nutrients. It is a significant factor.

## Understanding the micro nutrients that are found in food derived from animals.

Various micronutrients that are necessary for human health can be obtained from foods derived from animals. Here are some key micronutrients found in animal products and their functions:

**Vitamin B12:** Primarily found in meat, fish, eggs, and dairy, vitamin B12 is crucial for nerve function, DNA synthesis, and red blood cell formation.

**Iron:** Red meat, poultry, and fish are rich sources of

heme iron, which is more easily absorbed by the body compared to non-heme iron found in plant foods. Iron is essential for oxygen transport in the blood and energy metabolism.

**Zinc:** Present in meat, shellfish, and poultry, zinc plays a role in immune function, wound healing, and DNA synthesis.

**Calcium:** Although commonly associated with dairy products, calcium is also found in smaller amounts in canned fish with bones (such as sardines and salmon). Calcium is essential for the maintenance of bones, the functioning of muscles, and the transmission of nerves.

**Vitamin D:** Fatty fish like salmon, mackerel, and tuna are excellent sources of vitamin D, which is essential for the absorption of calcium, bone health, and immune function.

**Omega-3 fatty acids:** Found predominantly in fatty fish like salmon, trout, and sardines, omega-3s are important for heart health, brain function, and reducing inflammation.

**Vitamin A:** Liver, dairy products, and eggs are good sources of preformed vitamin A, important for vision, immune function, and skin health.

**Choline:** Present in eggs, liver, and poultry, choline is important for brain development, nerve function, and metabolism.

It's important to include a variety of animal-based foods in the diet to ensure adequate intake of these micronutrients. However, it's also essential to balance them with plant-based foods to obtain a wide array of nutrients and to minimize the intake of saturated fats and cholesterol often found in animal products.

## **Health Benefits of Animal-Based Nutrition**

Animal-based nutrition can provide several health benefits due to the rich array of nutrients they contain like.

Improved muscle growth and repair

Enhanced cognitive function

Better absorption of nutrients etc.

Some of the key benefits include:

**High-Quality Protein:** Animal products like meat, fish, eggs, and dairy are excellent sources of high-quality protein, which is crucial for building and repairing tissues, maintaining muscle mass, and supporting immune function.

**Essential Nutrients:** Animal foods are rich in essential nutrients such as vitamin B12, which is primarily found in animal products and essential for nerve function and DNA synthesis. They also provide heme iron, a highly absorbable form of iron important for preventing anemia.

**Omega-3 Fatty Acids:** Fatty fish like salmon, mackerel, and sardines are rich in omega-3 fatty acids, which have been associated with numerous health benefits, including reducing inflammation, supporting heart health, and promoting brain function.

**Vitamin D:** Certain animal products, such as fatty fish, egg yolks, and fortified dairy, are good sources of vitamin D, which is essential for bone know health, immune function, and overall well-being.

**Complete Amino Acid Profile:** Animal proteins generally contain all essential amino acids in the right proportions, making them "complete" proteins that support various bodily functions, including enzyme production, hormone regulation, and tissue repair.

**Satiety:** Animal products are often more satiating than plant-based foods, which can help with weight management by reducing overall calorie intake and preventing overeating.

While animal-based nutrition offers these benefits, it's essential to consume them as part of a balanced diet that also includes plenty of fruits, vegetables, whole grains, and healthy fats to ensure optimal health and nutrition. Additionally, sourcing animal products from sustainable and ethically-raised sources is crucial for both personal health and the environment.

## *Clarifying the role of animal products in a balanced diet*

Animal products can play a role in a balanced diet as they provide essential nutrients such as high-quality protein, vitamin B12, iron, zinc, and omega-3 fatty acids. However, it's important to consume them in moderation and to choose lean sources to minimize saturated fat intake. For those who choose not to consume animal products, it's possible to obtain these nutrients from plant-based sources with careful planning. Ultimately, a balanced diet should include a variety of foods from different sources to ensure adequate nutrient intake.

# CHAPTER 2
# ENHANCING ANIMAL-BASED DIETARY INTAKE FOR PARTICULAR HEALTH OBJECTIVES.

Choosing nutrient-rich animal products that support your goals is the first step in optimizing animal-based nutrition for particular health objectives. Lean meats, such as chicken breast or fish, are high in protein and can help build muscle. Oily fish is a good source of omega-3 fatty acids for heart health. You can also optimize your consumption of eggs for brain function or dairy for bone health. It's critical to strike a balance between these decisions and moderation and variety in your diet overall. Speaking with a nutritionist or dietitian can help you receive individualized advice based on your unique needs and health goals.

# Body composition and weight control

Foods derived from animals can improve body composition and help control weight in a number of ways.

**High Protein Content:** Foods derived from animals, including fish, poultry, eggs, dairy, and lean meats, are high in protein. Protein is well-known for its ability to promote a healthy body composition by lowering hunger, increasing satiety, and preserving lean muscle mass while losing weight.

**Nutrient Density:** Diets derived from animals offer vital nutrients that are critical for metabolism and general health, such as iron and zinc, as well as vitamins (like vitamin D and B vitamins). Eating foods high in nutrients can assist in maintaining energy levels and metabolism while controlling weight.

**Thermic Effect of Food (TEF):** The metabolism of protein requires more energy than that of fats and carbohydrates because protein has a higher TEF. This may help with weight management by slightly raising caloric expenditure.

**Muscle Growth and Maintenance:** All of the essential amino acids required for muscle growth and maintenance are found in protein sources derived from animals. Sustaining muscle mass during weight loss is essential for sustaining metabolic rate and encouraging a healthy body composition.

Foods derived from animals, particularly those rich in protein and good fats, can help boost feelings of fullness and satisfaction, which can lower overall calorie intake and support weight management objectives.

But it's crucial to include foods derived from animals in a balanced diet, along with lots of fruits, vegetables, whole grains, and healthy fats. Additionally, you can make sure you're getting the nutrients you need without consuming excessive amounts of saturated fat and cholesterol by selecting lean cuts of meat and incorporating a variety of protein sources. Before making big dietary changes, always get advice from a medical professional or registered dietitian, particularly if you have any particular health issues or dietary restrictions.

## *Athletic performance and recuperation*

Because animal-based nutrition contains high-quality protein, essential amino acids, and nutrients like iron and zinc that are bioavailable, it can have a substantial impact on athletic performance and recovery. In addition to providing the building blocks for muscle growth and repair, foods like lean meats, poultry, fish, eggs, and dairy products also support immune system function and energy metabolism. Athletes can improve their post-exercise recovery and maximize their performance by including these foods in a balanced diet.

## Benefits of eating an animal-based diet for sports performance and recuperation

Animal-based diets have a number of advantages for athletic performance and recuperation:

**High-quality protein:** can be found in abundance in animal-based diets, including lean meats, chicken, fish, eggs, and dairy products. These foods also contain all of the essential amino acids required for the growth and repair of muscles. Sufficient consumption of protein promotes muscle repair and training adaptation, which enhances performance.

**Creatine:** a substance found in some animal-based diets, such as fish and beef, helps supply energy for muscle contractions during intense exercise. It has been demonstrated that giving athletes creatine supplements increases their strength, power, and muscle mass.

**Bioavailability of Nutrients:** Compared to plant sources, animal-based diets frequently include nutrients like iron, zinc, vitamin B12, and omega-3 fatty acids in forms that are easier for the body to absorb and use. These nutrients are essential for immune system function, energy metabolism, oxygen transport, and inflammation regulation—all of which are necessary for optimum athletic performance and recuperation.

**Heme Iron:** Heme iron comes from animal sources and is more readily absorbed by the body than non-heme iron, which is present in plant-based diets. Sufficient levels of iron are necessary for the best possible oxygen delivery to working muscles, which helps to avoid fatigue and promote recovery.

**Growth Factors:** Whey protein and insulin-like growth factor 1 (IGF-1) are two growth factors found in dairy products that may aid in the synthesis of muscle proteins and the healing process after exercise.

**Satiety and Weight Management:** Eating foods derived from animals, especially those rich in protein and good fats, can help athletes maintain a healthy body composition, which is crucial for both performance and recuperation.

**Taste and Palatability:** Foods derived from animals frequently have a pleasant taste and texture, making them a fun addition to a diet for athletes. This can promote general dietary adherence and guarantee adherence to nutrition plans.

While eating a diet high in animal products can help athletes perform better and recuperate faster, each person has different needs and preferences. In order to meet nutrient requirements, support general health, and enhance athletic performance, a balanced diet comprising a variety of foods derived from both plants and animals is usually advised. When choosing a diet, ethical, environmental, and health-related factors should also be taken into account.

# Taking care of long-term illnesses with food decisions based on animal nutrition

Making dietary decisions to manage chronic conditions—with an emphasis on animal-based nutrition in particular—requires careful thought. Although diets based on animals can supply vital nutrients, it's crucial to pay attention to the kinds and quantities of food taken in order to promote general health and properly treat chronic illnesses.

## *Below are some general principles to consider:*

**Quality of Animal Products:** Choose fish that is high in omega-3 fatty acids, skinless chicken, and lean meat cuts. Select dairy products that are minimal in added sugars and saturated fats.

**Portion Control:** Eat in moderation to prevent consuming too many calories, which can aggravate chronic illnesses like diabetes and heart disease and cause weight gain.

**Balanced Macronutrients:** Try to have the right amounts of healthy fats, carbohydrates, and protein at each meal. While plant-based sources of protein, such as legumes and nuts, offer diversity and extra nutrients, animal protein can also contribute to the maintenance of muscle health.

**Reduce Your Consumption of Processed Meats:** Because processed meats, like bacon, sausage, and deli meats, are frequently high in saturated fats and sodium, they raise your risk of developing cardiovascular disease and other chronic illnesses.

**Emphasis on Whole Foods:** Include in your diet whole, minimally processed foods like dairy, fruits, vegetables, lean meats, fish, eggs, and whole grains. Essential nutrients and fiber from these foods support general health and may aid in the management of long-term conditions like diabetes and hypertension.

**Customized Approach:** Consult a medical professional or registered dietitian to customize your diet to meet your unique health requirements and dietary preferences. They can assist you in developing a customized meal plan that takes into consideration your lifestyle choices, nutritional needs, and chronic conditions.

To effectively manage chronic conditions, it is important to prioritize overall dietary balance and moderation, even though animal-based nutrition can have a place in a healthy diet. Along with dietary decisions, maintaining a healthy weight and continuing to be physically active are also essential for managing chronic conditions.

# CHAPTER 3
# IMPLEMENTING AN ANIMAL-BASED DIET.

Eating primarily animal products—meat, fish, eggs, and dairy—is the foundation of an animal-based diet. Here are some actions to think about:

**Plan your meals:** Make animal-based proteins, such as fish, poultry, and eggs, the main focus of your meals. If desired, add dairy products like yogurt, cheese, and milk.

**Incorporate Healthy Fats:** Diets centered around animals inherently comprise beneficial fats such as monounsaturated fats found in meat and omega-3 fatty acids found in fish.

**Variety Is Essential:** Eat a range of foods derived from animals to make sure you're getting a variety of nutrients. Incorporate seafood, fish, poultry, and red meat into your diet.

**Watch Portion Sizes:** Be mindful of portion sizes to prevent consuming excessive amounts of calories and saturated fats, which may cause health problems.

**Maintain a Balance with Vegetables:** Don't overlook vegetables in favor of animal-based diets. They offer vital fiber, vitamins, and minerals to promote general health.

**Stay Hydrated:** If you eat a diet high in protein-rich foods, it's important to stay hydrated by drinking lots of water throughout the day.

**Speak with an expert:** To make sure you're fulfilling your nutritional needs, think about speaking with a registered dietitian or nutritionist if you're making big dietary changes.

Always pay attention to what your body is telling you and modify your diet accordingly.

Useful advice on increasing the amount of animal-based foods in your diet

*You can increase the amount of animal-based foods in your diet in a sustainable and well-balanced manner. Here are a few useful pointers:*

**Begin Gradually:** When incorporating more animal-based foods into your diet, begin with modest serving sizes and work your way up to larger ones over time.

**Select Reputable Sources:** Whenever possible, choose premium, ethically sourced animal products. Seek out labels indicating grass-fed, pasture-raised, or organic.

**Include Variety:** To guarantee a varied nutrient intake, include a range of animal-based foods, including lean meats, poultry, fish, eggs, dairy, and even organ meats.

**Balance with Plants:** To maintain overall balance and nutrition, increase your intake of animal-based foods while ensuring that you still get plenty of fruits, vegetables, whole grains, and legumes in your diet.

**Be Aware of Portion Sizes:** Be mindful of portion sizes to prevent consuming too many animal-based foods, which can have negative health effects. Try to eat in moderation and in a balanced manner.

**Try Different Cooking Techniques:** To keep your meals flavorful and interesting, experiment with different cooking techniques like grilling, baking, roasting, or steaming.

**Incorporate Good Fats:** Go for animal-based diets high in omega-3 fatty acids, which are present in fatty fish, and think about using avocado or olive oil for cooking when preparing meals.

**Speak with a Nutritionist:** A registered dietitian or nutritionist can assist you in creating a balanced diet that includes more foods derived from animals if you have any specific dietary requirements or health concerns.

Keep in mind that each person has unique nutritional requirements, so you must determine what is best for your body.

## Keeping an eye on cholesterol and other health indicators when feeding animals.

Regular blood testing is necessary to monitor lipid levels, such as total cholesterol, LDL (low-density lipoprotein), HDL (high-density lipoprotein), and triglycerides, in an animal-based diet. A complete picture of overall health can also be obtained by monitoring additional health markers like blood pressure, inflammation markers, and glucose levels. Seeking advice from a medical expert or dietitian can assist in interpreting these findings and, if required, modifying the diet to support ideal health.

## Methods of preservation for food based on animals

Food made from animals is usually preserved by freezing, canning, smoking, pickling, drying, or refrigeration. The particular steps and considerations for each method vary based on the kind of animal-based food you're preserving. As an illustration:

*Refrigeration:* Store foods derived from animals, such as fish, poultry, meat, and dairy products, in a refrigerator that is kept at or below 40°F (4°C).

*Freezing:* Before freezing at 0°F (-18°C) or lower, package meat, poultry, fish, and other animal-based foods in airtight containers or freezer bags.

*Drying:* Use a food dehydrator or a low-temperature oven to dry out meats or fish. The dried goods should be kept in a dry, cool environment in airtight containers.

*Smoking:* To enhance flavor and preserve meats and fish, use a smoker. When smoking, make sure the food reaches a safe internal temperature, and then store it appropriately.

*Curing:* To extract moisture and stop bacteria from growing, season meats with salt, sugar, and occasionally nitrites. Safe meat curing requires adhering to certain recipes and instructions.

*Pickling:* Marinate foods derived from animals, such as fish, eggs, or even meats, by immersing them in a brine solution that is made up of salt, vinegar, and spices. The pickled goods should be kept in the refrigerator in sterilized jars.

*Canning:* For acidic foods like pickled fish or meat, use traditional water bath canning techniques. For other foods, process meats, poultry, and fish in pressure canners. To guarantee safety, stick to approved canning techniques and tried-and-true recipes.

When preserving animal-based foods, always adhere to food safety regulations, including correct handling, storage, and hygiene practices, to avoid foodborne illnesses.

# CHAPTER 4
## MEAL PREPARATION AND RECIPE SUGGESTIONS FOR FOODS DERIVED FROM ANIMALS:

### *For breakfast:*

***Eggs:*** Try a veggie omelette or scrambled eggs with feta cheese and spinach.
Berries, Greek yogurt, and honey drizzled over.
Toast with avocado and bacon.

***Lunch:*** Caesar salad made with grilled chicken and homemade dressing.
Whole wheat pita pockets filled with tuna salad, tomatoes, and lettuce.

Brown rice and mixed vegetables are stir-fried with beef.

***Dinner:*** is Roasted asparagus and quinoa are served with baked salmon topped with a lemon-dill sauce.
Bacon or crispy pancetta paired with a creamy carbonara sauce.
Steamed broccoli and grilled steak served with garlic-mashed potatoes.

***Munchies:***
Cherry tomatoes and sliced cucumbers with cottage cheese.
Turkey slices from the deli are wrapped in cheese sticks.
Hard-boiled eggs seasoned with pepper and salt.

***Sweets:***
Greek yogurt parfait topped with granola and layers of fresh fruit.
Strawberries dipped in chocolate.
Homemade vanilla custard with a variety of berries on top.
For a well-rounded diet, don't forget to balance your meals with a range of fruits, vegetables, whole grains, and lean proteins.

# <u>20 recipe suggestions regarding food derived from animals</u>

Twenty recipe and meal planning ideas centered on animal-based foods:

***Chicken Parmesan:*** Marinara sauce, melted mozzarella cheese, and baked, breaded, and roasted chicken breasts served over spaghetti.

***Beef Tacos:*** Tortillas stuffed with seasoned ground beef, salsa, sour cream, cheese, and lettuce. Cooked with taco seasoning.

***Salmon Teriyaki:*** Rice and steamed vegetables are served with grilled or baked salmon fillets coated in teriyaki sauce.

***Vegetable Beef Stew:*** Flavorful broth simmers tender beef chunks with potatoes, carrots, onions, and celery.

Turkey chili is made with ground turkey, kidney beans, tomatoes, onions, and seasonings. It can be eaten over rice or with cornbread.

***Shrimp Scampi:*** Linguine tossed with sautéed shrimp, garlic, lemon juice, white wine, and parsley.

***Pork Tenderloin with Apples:*** This dish consists of roasted pork tenderloin, sautéed apples, onions, and mashed potatoes on the side.

***Stir-fried steak and broccoli:*** Thinly sliced beef is cooked alongside crunchy broccoli florets in a flavorful sauce and served over noodles or rice.

***A salad consisting of*** grilled chicken breast slices, romaine lettuce, croutons, Parmesan cheese, and Caesar dressing is called a chicken Caesar salad.

***Sandwiches with slow-cooked*** pulled pork mixed with barbecue sauce and served with coleslaw on buns.

***Roasted whole chicken*** with lemon, garlic, and herbs, accompanied by roasted potatoes and green beans, is known as lemon herb roast chicken.

***Sausage and Peppers:*** Marinara sauce, bell peppers, and onions are sautéed Italian sausages that are then served over pasta or in rolls.

***Shepherd's pie with ground beef:*** ground beef cooked in a rich gravy with vegetables, covered in mashed potatoes, and baked until golden.

***Honey Mustard Glazed Ham:*** Roasted vegetables are served alongside baked ham covered in a sweet and tangy honey mustard glaze.

***Creamy risotto cooked*** with soft chicken chunks, mushrooms, and Parmesan cheese is called chicken and mushroom risotto.

***Ground beef*** that has been spiced and served over rice with black beans, corn, avocado, salsa, and shredded cheese is called a beef burrito bowl.

***Pasta with Lemon Garlic Shrimp:*** Shrimp cooked with white wine, garlic, and zest, combined with pasta and fresh herbs.

***Chicken Piccata:*** thinly sliced chicken breasts cooked with mashed potatoes or pasta and capers in a lemon butter sauce.

***Chili con carne:*** tasty chili prepared from ground beef, kidney beans, onions, tomatoes, and a mixture of spices.

***Bacon-***Wrapped Stuffed Chicken Breast: Baked until golden and crispy, chicken breasts packed with cheese and spinach are covered in bacon.

To ensure that your meals are engaging and fulfilling, these recipes provide a range of flavors and cooking techniques.

# CHAPTER 5
# 101 FOODS ARE DERIVED FROM ANIMALS.

Chicken breast: these is highly protenious and has less fat

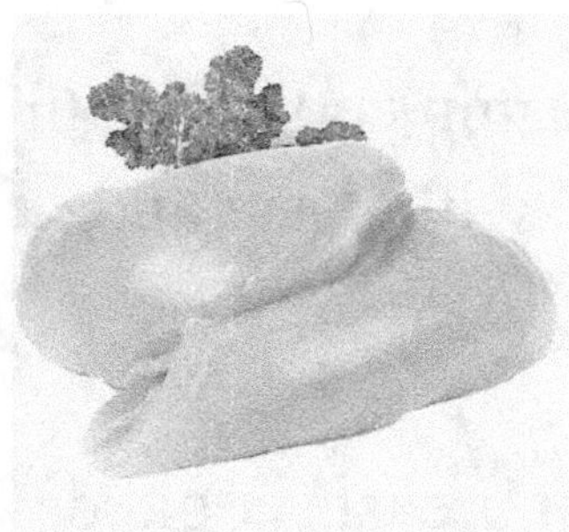

Salmon are plentiful in Omega-3 fatty acids and protein

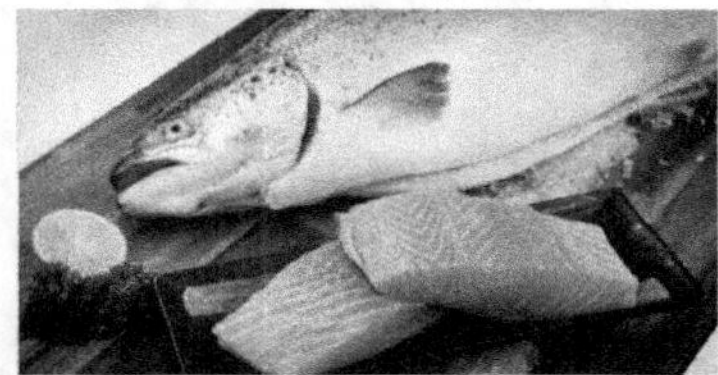

Eggs are a good source of vitamins, minerals, and protein.

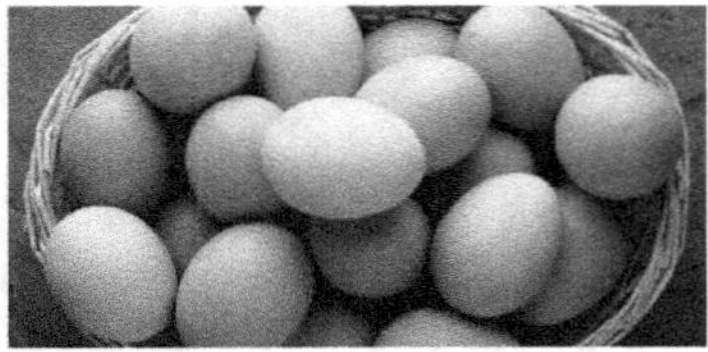

Protein, iron, and a variety of vitamins and minerals can all be found in beef.

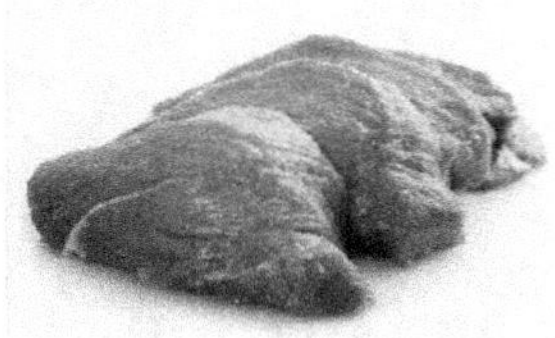

MILK: CONTAINS Vitamins D and B12, calcium, and protein

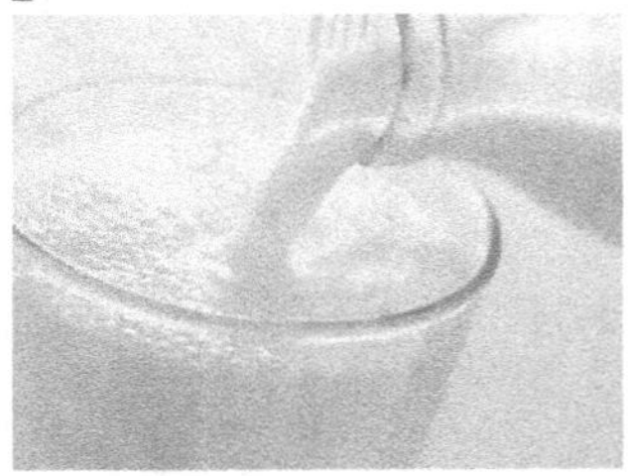

Yogurt: Probiotics, protein, calcium, and vitamins

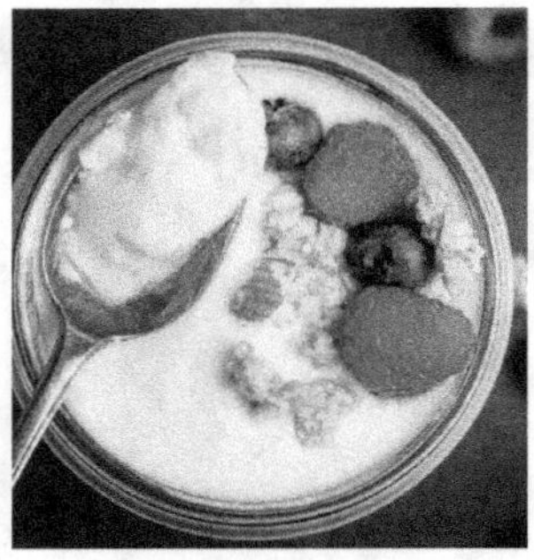

Cheese: packed with vitamins, protein, and calcium.

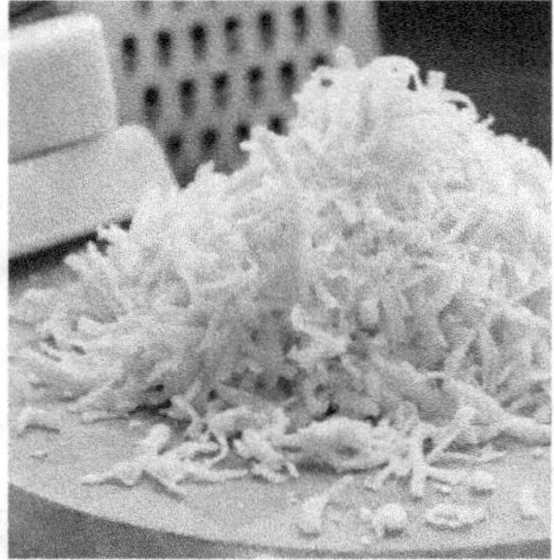

Shrimp is rich in protein, low in calories, and high in omega-3 fatty acids.

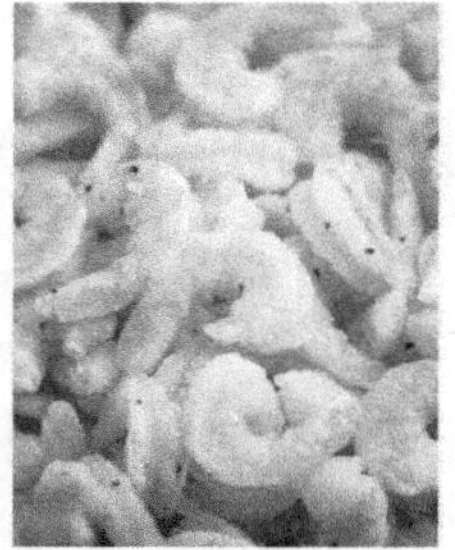

Turkey is a lean protein, vitamin, and mineral source.

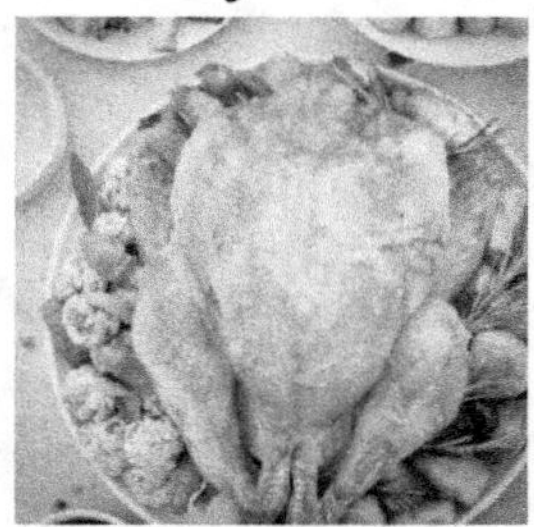

Pork provides minerals like phosphorus and zinc, as well as protein and B vitamins.

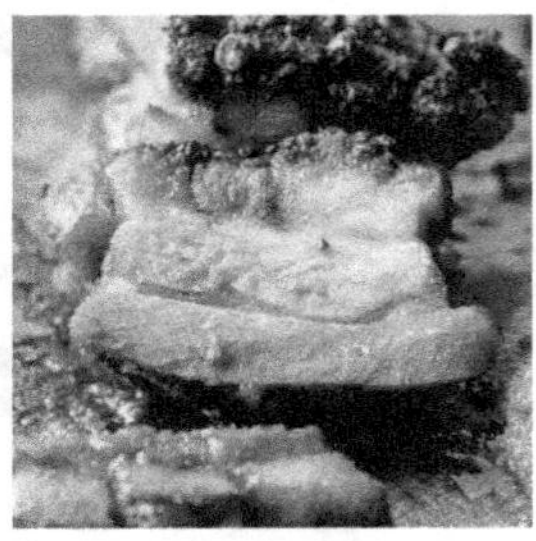

Lamb: iron, zinc, vitamin B12, protein, and selenium.

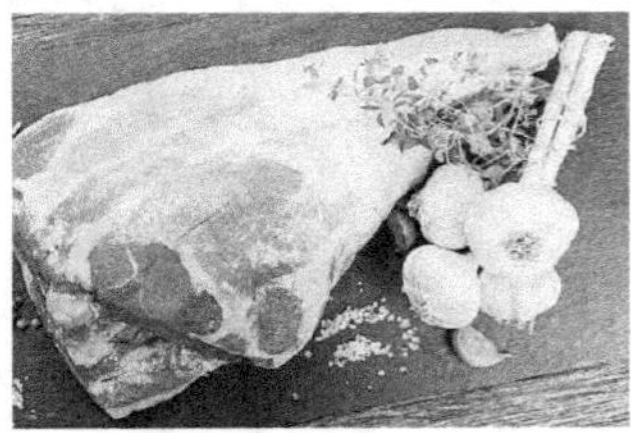

Duck: phosphorus, vitamin B6, niacin, iron, zinc, and

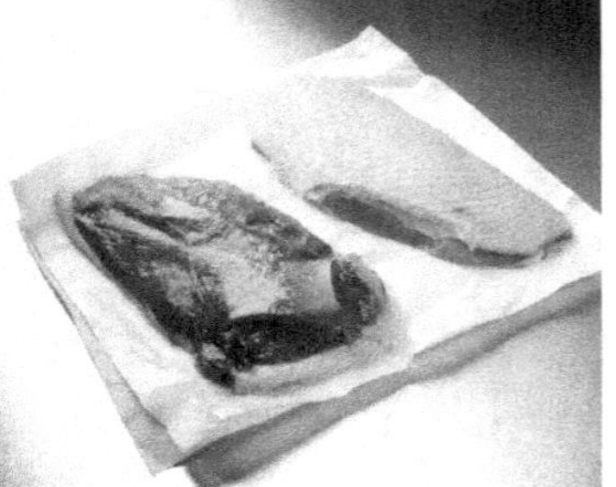

protein.

Quail: phosphorus, vitamin B12, iron, zinc, and protein.

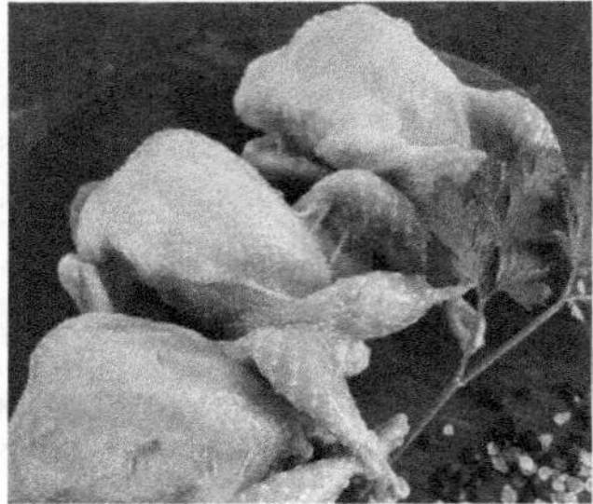

Rabbit: iron, zinc, B12, phosphorus, protein.

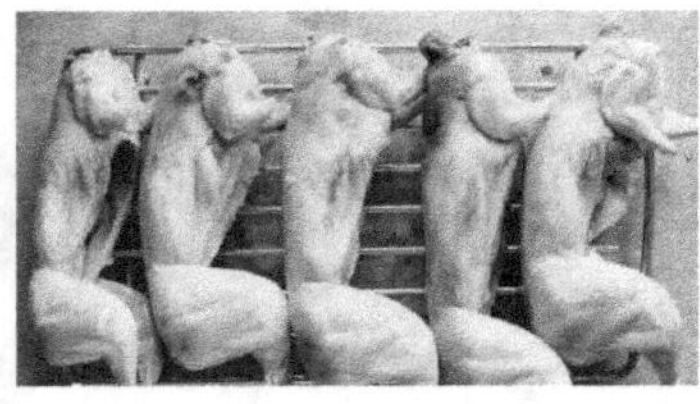

Venison: iron, zinc, vitamin B12, phosphorus, niacin, and protein.

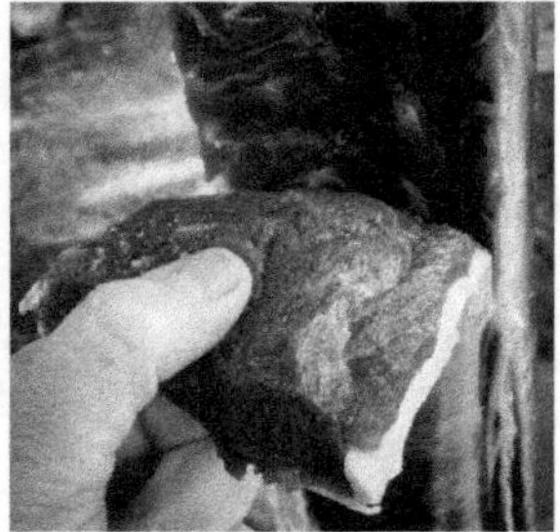

Bison: niacin, vitamin B12, iron, zinc, protein, and selenium.

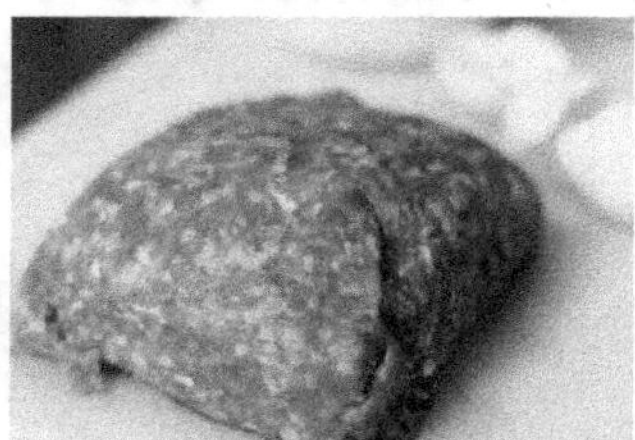

Goose: niacin, vitamin B12, protein, iron, zinc, and phosphorus.

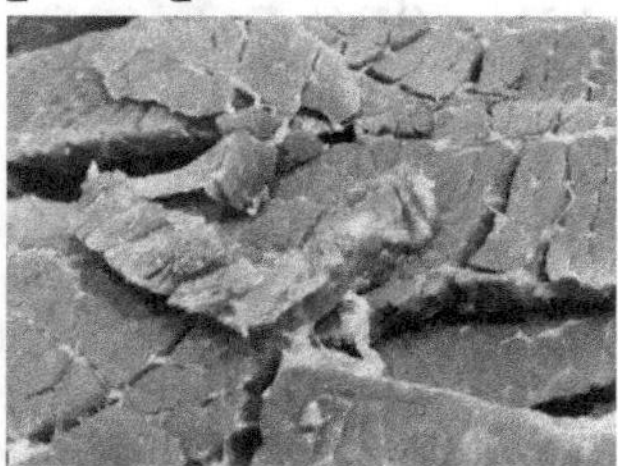

Veal: phosphorus, vitamin B12, iron, zinc, and protein.

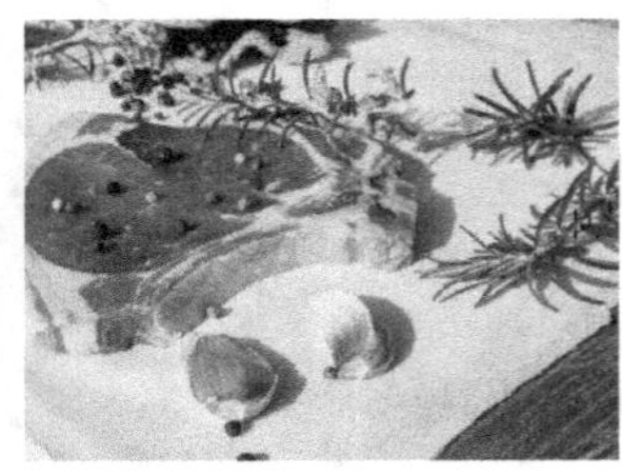

# CHAPTER 6

# Fish: protein, vitamin B12, vitamin D, selenium, iodine, and omega-3 fatty acids.

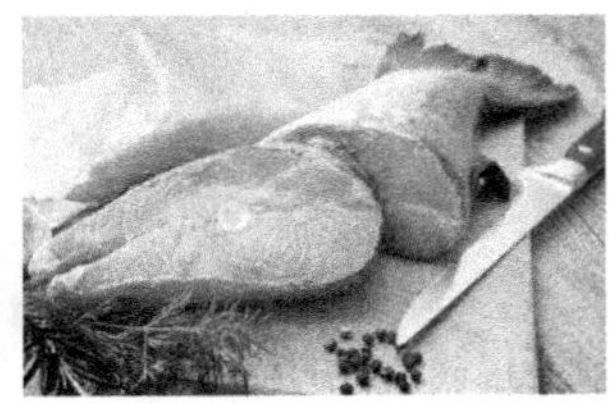

Vitamin D, B12, selenium, protein, and omega-3 fatty acids are all present in tuna.

Vitamin B12, vitamin D, protein, and omega-3 fatty acids are all present in trout.

Protein, omega-3 fatty acids, vitamin B12, vitamin D, and phosphorus are found in cod.

Haddock: vitamin B12, vitamin D, selenium, protein, and omega-3 fatty acids.

Hake: Vitamin D, B12, phosphorus, protein, and omega-3 fatty acids.

Halibut contains protein, vitamin B12, vitamin D, omega-3 fatty acids, and selenium.

Mackerel contains protein, vitamin B12, vitamin D, omega-3 fatty acids, and selenium.

Sardines: calcium, vitamin B12, vitamin D, protein, and omega-3 fatty acids.

Anchovies: protein, vitamin B12, vitamin D, selenium, and omega-3 fatty acids.

Vitamin D, B12, selenium, protein, and omega-3 fatty acids are all found in catfish.

Tilapia: phosphorus, selenium, protein, and vitamin B12.

Crab: copper, zinc, vitamin B12, protein.

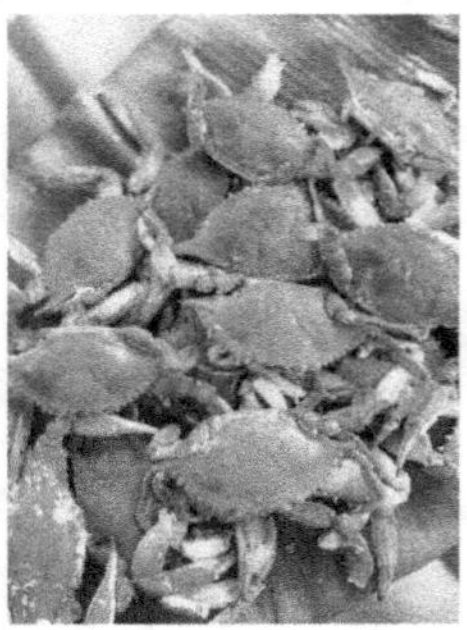

Lobster: copper, selenium, vitamin B12, and protein.

Protein, potassium, magnesium, and vitamin B12 make up scallops.

Clam: iron, zinc, protein, and vitamin B12.

Oyster: zinc, copper, vitamin B12, and protein.

Mussels: iron, manganese, protein, and vitamin B12.

Squid: copper, selenium, protein, and vitamin B12.

Octopus: iron, zinc, protein, and vitamin B12.

Protein, iron, magnesium, vitamin E, and snails (escargot).

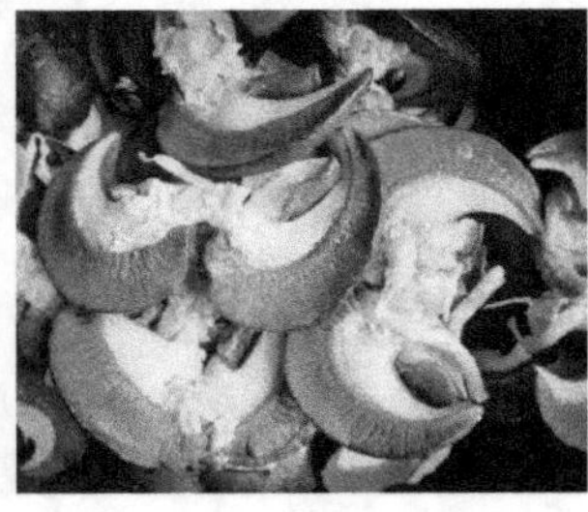

Legs of frogs: potassium, phosphorus, vitamin B12, protein.

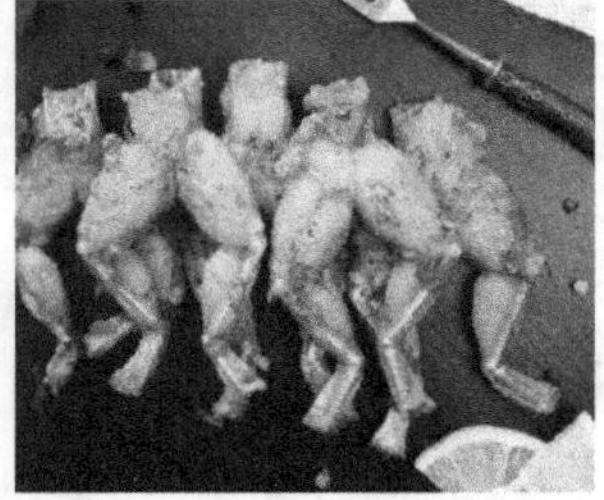

Alligator: Iron, zinc, protein, and vitamin B12.
Turtle: Niacin, protein, vitamin B12, and selenium.

Bison: iron, zinc, vitamin B12, and protein.

Elk: Iron, zinc, protein, and B12.

Rat kangaroo: iron, zinc, protein, and vitamin B12.

Emu: Iron, zinc, protein, and B12.

Pheasant: Niacin, phosphorus, selenium, protein.

Partridge: Iron, phosphorus, protein, and niacin.

Wild boar: zinc, niacin, thiamine, and protein.

Goat: Meat that is lean and rich in B vitamins, iron, zinc, and protein.

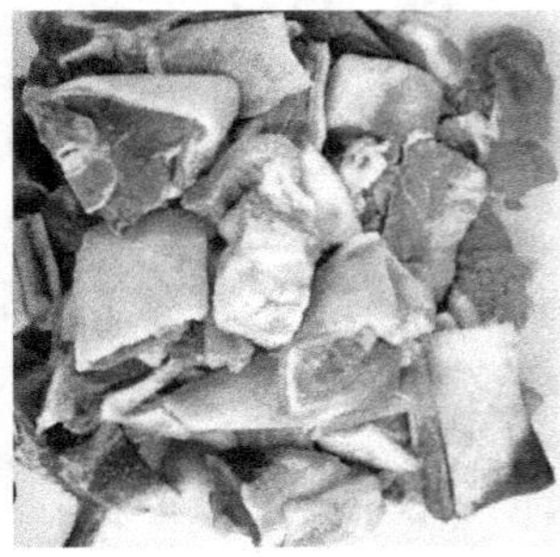

Venison: Rich in protein, iron, and B vitamins, but low in fat.

Buffalo: Full of protein, iron, zinc, and B vitamins; similar to beef but frequently leaner.

Ostrich meat is extremely lean, high in protein, low in fat, and high in B vitamins and iron.

Horse: Highly protein-rich, lean meat with iron, zinc, and B vitamins, comparable to beef.

Reindeer meat is lean and low in fat, high in protein, iron, and B vitamins.

Bear: Rich in iron, zinc, and B vitamins; also high in protein and fat.

Raccoon: Rich in iron and B vitamins, high in protein and fat.

Moose meat is lean and rich in B vitamins, iron, zinc, and protein.

Antelope: Iron and B vitamin-rich, lean meat with a high protein content that resembles venison.

Camel: Iron and B vitamins are among the important vitamins and minerals found in this lean, high-protein meat.

Yak: High in protein, iron, zinc, and B vitamins; comparable to beef.

Zebra: Protein-rich lean meat that also contains iron, vitamins, and minerals.

Eel: Packed with protein, calcium, phosphorus, vitamins A and D, and omega-3 fatty acids.

Swordfish: Rich in vitamin D, selenium, omega-3 fatty acids, and protein.

# CHAPTER 7
# MAHI-MAHI

Mahi-mahi: this fish is also high in protein, omega-3 fatty acids, and a variety of vitamins and minerals, including selenium and b vitamins.

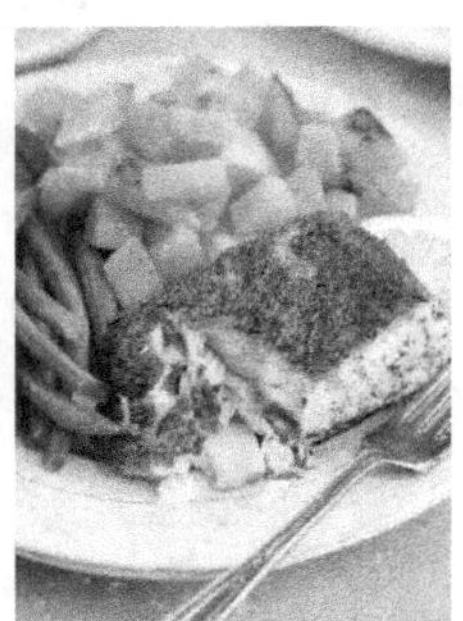

Omega-3 fatty acids, vitamin D, and protein are all abundant in kingfish.

Omega-3 fatty acids, vitamins B6 and B12, and minerals like magnesium and selenium are all found in grouper, which is high in protein.

Omega-3 fatty acids, B vitamins, and protein are all found in good amounts in catfish.

Omega-3 fatty acids, protein, and a variety of vitamins and minerals are all abundant in perch.

Lean white fish high in protein, omega-3 fatty acids, and different vitamins and minerals is called Pollock.

Flounder: A lean white fish that is high in protein, omega-3 fatty acids, and important nutrients. It resembles Pollock.

Sole: Rich in protein, vitamins B12 and D, and minerals like phosphorus and selenium, sole is a great food choice.

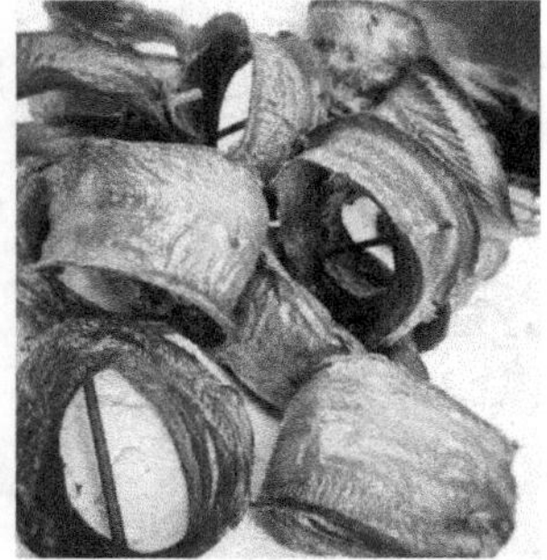

Herring: Omega-3 fatty acids, which are abundant in herring, are good for heart health. Moreover, it offers protein, vitamin B12, and vitamin D.

Monkfish: Rich in minerals like phosphorus and selenium, monkfish is also a good source of lean protein and contains the vitamins B6 and B12.

Omega-3 fatty acids, protein, vitamin D, and vitamin B12 are all found in abundance in bluefish.

Amberjack: Omega-3 fatty acids, vitamins B6 and B12, and protein are all abundant in amberjack.

Mullet: This fish is high in protein, omega-3 fatty acids, and a number of vitamins and minerals, such as calcium, iron, and vitamin A.

Pompano: Rich in protein, omega-3 fatty acids, and vitamins B6 and B12, pompano is a great vegetable.

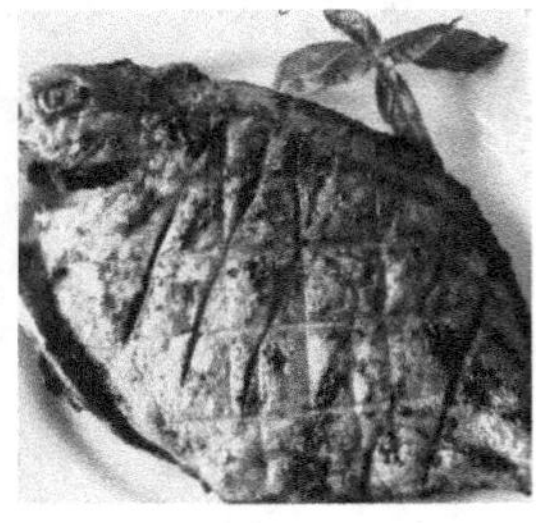

Redfish: Rich in vitamin B12, vitamin D, omega-3 fatty acids, and protein.

Wahoo: Rich in omega-3 fatty acids, protein, and vitamins B6 and B12.

Omega-3 fatty acids, potassium, selenium, vitamins B12 and D, and protein are all abundant in triggerfish.

Mahi-mahi: Rich in protein, low in fat, and an excellent source of niacin, phosphorus, selenium, and vitamins B6 and B12.

Fish roe, or caviar, is rich in protein, vitamin B12, vitamin D, selenium, and omega-3 fatty acids.

Duck or goose liver, or foie grass, is rich in iron, copper, zinc, choline, vitamin A, and vitamin B12. Plus, it has a lot of fat.

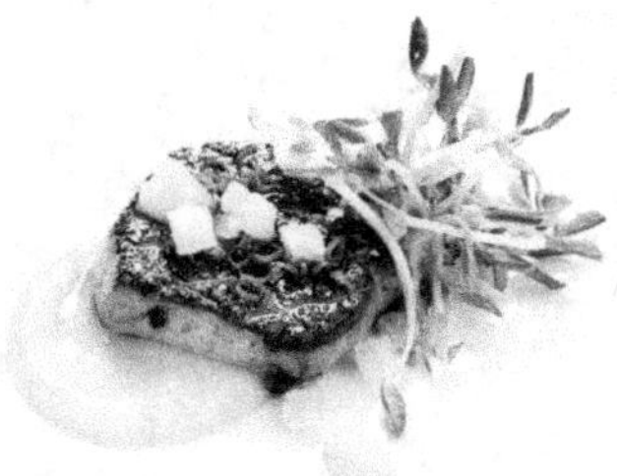

A wonderful source of protein, iron, magnesium, selenium, and vitamin B12 is escargot, or snails.

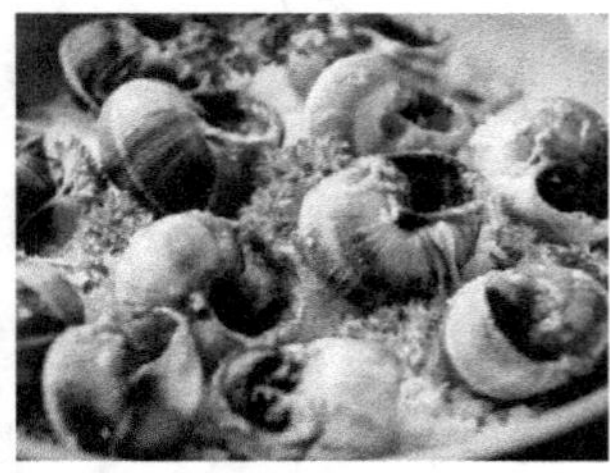

Bone marrow: Packed with protein, iron, vitamins A and K, fatty acids, and healthy fats, especially monounsaturated fats.

Chicken liver is rich in iron, folate, protein, and vitamins A and B12.

Beef liver is a nutrient-dense food that is high in iron, zinc, copper, selenium, vitamin A, and vitamin B12.

Vitamin B12, iron, zinc, and protein are all abundant in beef tongue.

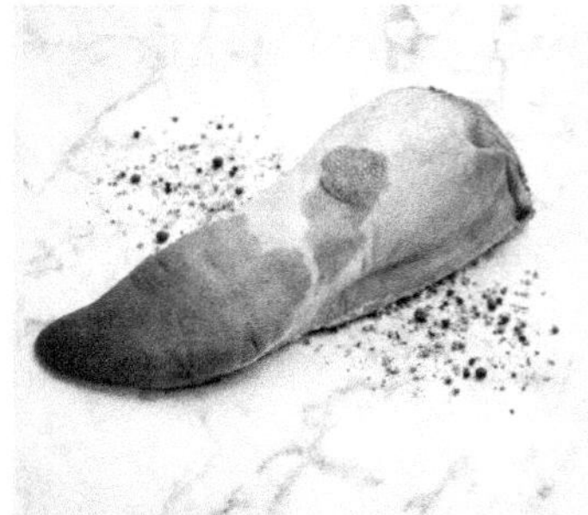

Chicken feet: Rich in collagen, these are good for skin elasticity and joint health.

Chicken gizzards are a great source of iron, zinc, phosphorus, and protein.

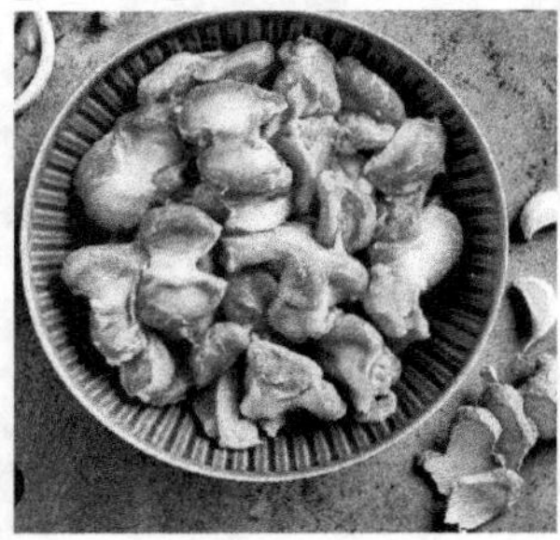

Tripe made from beef: Tripe is high in protein, zinc, selenium, and vitamin B12.

B vitamins, especially B12, iron, zinc, and protein are all abundant in chicken hearts.

Pig's ears: They have more fat than other options, but they also contain protein, fat, and a few vitamins and minerals.

Protein, iron, zinc, vitamin B12, riboflavin, niacin, and phosphorus are all found in pig feet.

Pork cheeks: Iron, zinc, protein, riboflavin, niacin, vitamin B12, and phosphorus.

Pork belly: phosphorus, riboflavin, niacin, iron, zinc, and vitamin B12.

Lamb sweetbreads: Iron, zinc, riboflavin, niacin, vitamin B12, phosphorus, and protein.

Pork liver contains protein, phosphorus, iron, zinc, vitamin B12, riboflavin, and niacin.

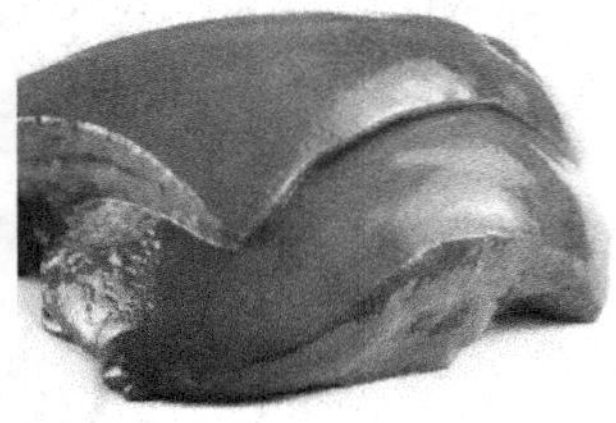

Pork kidney: Iron, zinc, riboflavin, niacin, phosphorus, protein, and vitamin B12.

Protein, Iron, Zinc, B12, Riboflavin, Niacin, and Phosphorus are all present in lamb kidneys.

Protein, Iron, Zinc, Vitamin B12, Riboflavin, Niacin, and Phosphorus are found in lamb brains.

Cod liver oil contains chicken eggs, vitamin D, vitamin A, vitamin E, and omega-3 fatty acids (EPA and DHA).

Quail eggs: Choline, protein, riboflavin, selenium, vitamin B12, and vitamin D.

These foods offer a variety of vital nutrients that are critical for maintaining general health, such as iron for oxygen transport, protein for muscle growth and repair, different vitamins for immunity and metabolism, and minerals for healthy bones and other body processes. By providing a variety of vital nutrients like protein, healthy fats, vitamins, and minerals, it can also support a balanced diet.

Essential nutrients found in meats include zinc for immune system function, iron for oxygen transport, protein for healthy muscles, and B vitamins for energy metabolism. However these meats can differ in terms of fat content, which impacts their calorie density and appropriateness for various dietary requirements.

## Conclusion

In the exploration of optimizing health through animal-based food, we've delved into the rich nutritional benefits and considerations surrounding this dietary approach. From the ancestral roots of relying on animal products for sustenance to the modern understanding of their role in supporting overall vitality, it's clear that these foods offer a plethora of essential nutrients crucial for well-being.

Throughout this discussion, we've highlighted the importance of quality sourcing and mindful consumption when incorporating animal-based foods into your diet. By choosing responsibly sourced options and prioritizing nutrient density, you can maximize the health-promoting benefits while minimizing potential ethical, environmental, and health concerns.

While the debate surrounding animal-based versus plant-based diets persists, it's essential to recognize that both approaches can coexist within a balanced dietary pattern. Whether you opt for a predominantly animal-based diet or choose to incorporate these foods alongside plant-based alternatives, the key lies in finding what works best for your individual needs and preferences.

Ultimately, optimizing your health with animal-based food is about making informed choices that prioritize both personal well-being and broader ethical and environmental considerations. By embracing a diverse array of nutrient-rich foods and listening to your body's cues, you can cultivate a dietary pattern that nourishes not only your physical health but also your overall vitality and longevity.

As you continue on your journey towards optimal health, may you find balance, satisfaction, and fulfillment in the nourishing power of animal-based foods, and may your dietary choices align with your values, preferences, and aspirations for a vibrant and thriving life.

www.ingramcontent.com/pod-product-compliance
Lightning Source LLC
Chambersburg PA
CBHW070733260726
48660CB00007B/2829